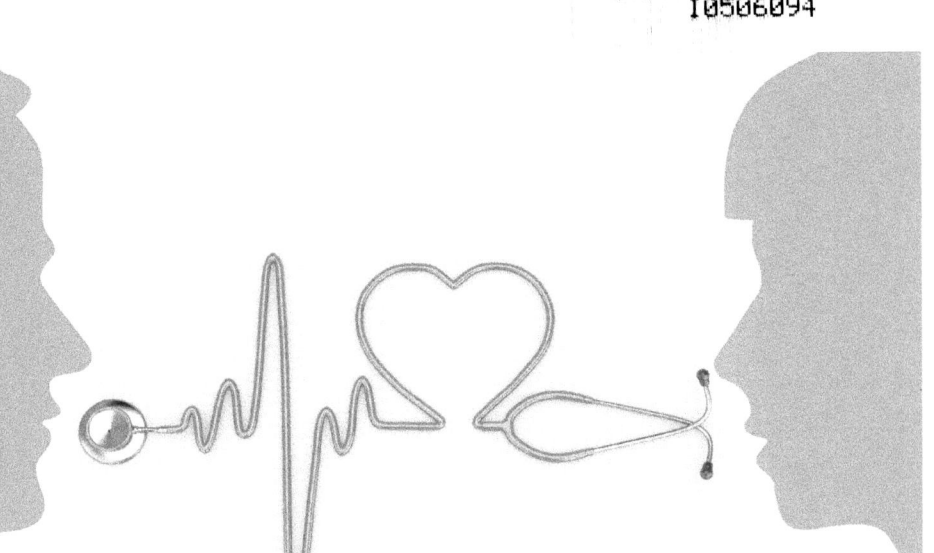

HEALING
Conversations

ESSENTIAL COMMUNICATIONS FOR HEALTHCARE PROFESSIONALS

8 Critical Conversations and
10 Simple Practices that Promote Patient Healing

ANN FITZGERALD PhD

Copyright © 2014 Ann Fitzgerald PhD
All rights reserved.

ISBN: 1494942313
ISBN 13: 9781494942311

Dedication

This book on the healing potential in conversations is dedicated to all patients—past, present, and future. Patients of the past have taught us what is meaningful and helpful during injury and illness. Patients that we currently work with provide the opportunity for us to connect as we may never have done before. Patients of the future will achieve greater healing as we caregivers apply our learning and refined skills to the conversations we have with them.

ACKNOWLEDGEMENT

Several important people in my life strongly influenced the writing of this book. My appreciation first goes to my wonderful husband, Bruce, whose frequent need to interact with the healthcare world over his last ten years of life taught me what really matters most to those who are anxious and ill; to my father and stepfather who both influenced my decision to pursue a healthcare career; to my brother, Ron, who has proven a wonderful caretaker for his wife, Marie, and the source for many patient-experience stories; to my beautiful, supportive, and talented daughters, Laurie Fitzgerald Tortorella and Ellyn Reynolds, who always insisted that there was a book in me; and finally to my wonderful friend and mentor Wendy Leebov for walking with me through the early stages of this book. I also appreciate the rich suggestions of my talented nursing colleagues and artful communicators Vicki Calvin, Karen English, Susan Marks, Sister Barbara Noble, and Joanne Law and the special review by writing coach T.L. Champion and patient-experience expert Jill Golde.

TABLE OF CONTENTS

Acknowledgement · v
Preface · ix
Introduction: Fundamentals of HEALING *Conversations* · · · · · · · · · · · · xv

Part I   Why Healthcare Communications Break Down   1
Chapter 1   So Many People! · 3
Chapter 2   The "Decide, Determine, and Direct" Mentality · · · · · · · · · · 9
Chapter 3   Unconscious Incompetence · 15
Chapter 4   The "Good is Good Enough" Mind-Set · · · · · · · · · · · · · · · · 19
Chapter 5   Anxiety at the Forefront · 23
Chapter 6   Patient Becomes a Diagnosis · 25

Part II Caregiver-Led Conversations: What Helps? What Heals? 29
Chapter 7   Let Me *Feel* Your Caring · 33
Chapter 8   Treat Me As *I Want* to Be Treated · · · · · · · · · · · · · · · · · · · 43
Chapter 9   Hear What I Don't Say · 47
Chapter 10 Let Me Know *What's What* · 51
Chapter 11 Help Me *Feel* Safe and Be Safe · 55
Chapter 12 Let Me Know I'll *Not Suffer* · 59
Chapter 13 Help Me *Help* My Family · 63
Chapter 14 Tell Me What I Want to Know,
            When I'm *Ready* to Hear It. · 67

**Part III Practices for Caregivers and Patients That Enhance
           Communication and Speed Healing   71**
Chapter 15 Caregiver Practices That Support
            HEALING *Conversations* · 73

Chapter 16 Patient Practices That Encourage
            HEALING *Conversations* ·81

CONCLUSION · 89
References ·91
Appendix: A Patient's Guide to HEALING Conversations · · · · · · · · · · ·93

PREFACE

Health care became my destiny a week short of my sixth birthday. Memories of the precise moment remain vivid.

The year is 1950 and the location is my home in East Petersburg, PA. My brother, Ron, and I huddle together in our dining room trying to sort out what is happening. Everything in our house seems out of sorts this night—unfamiliar. Something very important is happening but we don't know what. Our grandfather, who happens to be a minister, arrives at the front door, along with the family doctor. Our mother seems nervous, almost mysterious, as she ushers them upstairs. Everyone is talking in hushed tones. Aunt Marion keeps wringing her hands and retreating to the kitchen. Ron and I are told to stay downstairs. There is so much whispering. No one looks at my brother and me.

Ron, age ten, figures things out. He announces with a certainty that attests to his advanced age that our father just died. Neither of us is sure what this means. We don't know anyone who died. We just know that in that hour our world has changed—forever.

Dad was ill for years. This was before dialysis machines, and physicians had no big guns to help our father overcome his kidney disease. He stayed in bed for days on end. Home care nurses regularly came and went. His limited activity was our daily normal. My mother knew our father had but a year to live, but she thought this was her burden alone. Death and dying were not topics for children. No adult explained to us what had happened in our home that night. We were whisked off to our cousin's house until funeral arrangements were final.

My brother and I were confused as we witnessed tearful people streaming past our father's coffin at the church—and heard Aunt Arlene's loud sobs. We couldn't figure out why she was behaving this way. It was unsettling to see our mother cry. I was told I acted out. I don't know exactly what I did, but whatever it was, my unruly behavior exempted me from attending the graveside service.

I still recall palpable fear as we waited in the dining room that fateful night. When my brother told me Dad had died, a wave of sadness overwhelmed me. I became very frightened. My muddled thoughts turned to God. Why would God take away such a wonderful man as my father? Would I be next? What would stop God from having me die too? Consumed by fear, I bargained with God.

This is what I promised: I'll become a nurse and help others if you will just spare me. Let me live.

Flash forward to 1962, in a large academic medical center in Philadelphia.

I'm a student nurse about to get my very first patient assignment. I am dressed in a pristine white, aproned uniform, common student nurse garb for the era. I am so excited about going into a clinical area. Then comes crushing disappointment and dismay. My very first assignment: *talk* to the patient.

What? At eighteen, I did not find this an easy task. The patient was a stranger, he was sick, and he was older than my stepfather! What could we possibly have in common? And what could we possibly say?

I think often of the wisdom in that assignment. It remains as relevant today as it was back then. Speaking with patients and their families, although challenging, is essential to healing.

I wrote this book because for many years I have been and continue to be a caregivers' advocate. I understand just how hard it is to ensure that patients are safe, that they get the precise treatment and care they need, and that they get better as a result of all we do for them. And I want caregivers to be successful in their efforts. Along the way, my husband, Bruce, developed multiple chronic health problems that required years of medical care. I too eventually wound up in the patient role for several hospital admissions, so I know how important communications can be.

A majority of the time, Bruce's experiences and mine, as both a patient and spouse, were satisfactory. Most caregivers we met were kind and considerate. What was lacking in these encounters, however, was understanding. Some call it empathy. Who we were—what mattered most to us as individuals and as a family, what havoc illness was causing in our lives—these matters simply were not at the forefront, let alone documented in any care plan.

My passion for patients and families grew stronger and stronger as I realized that although everyone was working hard, most lacked the essential communications skills to deal with us effectively. They simply did not know how to tune in and care for us. Conversations did not move to dialogue, which would have included our perspective. Caregiver communications, in large part, lacked the healing factor.

Today, my goal is simple: help caregivers be successful in communicating with patients and families to promote greater healing. I am convinced that healing requires meaningful dialogue on practical and relevant matters, and this dialogue must be conducted in a sensitive and caring way. This is the essence of healing conversations. All engaged in patient care need communications savvy—we need to hold certain conversations and hold them well.

Here is the clinch. Many of us in healthcare—nurses, doctors, technologists, aides, and others—have little to no communications training. I am talking about instruction in the ability to engage in meaningful dialogue. And few patients, even those with high IQs or advanced education, know how to communicate effectively with healthcare workers, especially when illness, injury or high-stake wellness initiatives are involved.

Thus it is essential that as caregivers we take the lead—that we facilitate. Our attention needs to be focused on ways to convey genuine concern for each patient's experience. When we express concern, we allow relevant and important information to surface and get addressed.

Communication failures create a chasm between the patient and the caregiver. My childhood story of the night my father died, serves as a powerful example of a healing conversation simply not held.

In my student-nurse story, both the patient and I were at a loss for words. We were in a relationship in which we both were learning to speak. For me it was all about how I might best serve this patient. For the patient it was his knowing how to speak of things that were happening to him— his condition and his concerns about the likelihood that treatment would make him whole again. Neither of us was fluent in the language that would connect us. I had no preparation or foreknowledge of conversations that heal.

The quality of our conversations with patients has a powerful impact on the patient and family experience. Engaging in open dialogue—as well as having the skills to do so—is essential.

More about This Book

I'm writing this book for professional caregivers and healthcare students—of all types and ages. It also includes suggestions for when patients need to take initiative—to start or lead a conversation that is important to healing. Caregivers can give this helpful information to patients and their families, especially those dealing with long-term, chronic health issues.

The Introduction lays the foundation by exploring two core concepts: the relationship between patient and professional caregiver, and the role of communications in healing. Part I delineates the communication challenges inherent in health care. Part II features the CLEAR Communications model and eight conversations that are important to patients. Caregivers need to develop the skills to handle these conversations well. Quite simply, healing is impaired if these conversations are *not* held. Part III offers five communications practices that caregivers should embrace and five communication practices that are the responsibility of patients and families. The appendix features a handout that caregivers can provide to patients. This information cues patients and families so that they can do their part to ensure that the conversations between them and their caregivers are healing ones.

HEALING *Conversations* expresses my commitment to shine light on the communications that lie at the core of satisfying, heartwarming, and healing patient experiences.

INTRODUCTION: FUNDAMENTALS OF HEALING CONVERSATIONS

The dynamics of the care relationship and the role of communications in healing affect the patient's experience and outcomes.

The Patient-Caregiver Relationship

The relationship between caregiver and patient is special. This human connection is critical to restoration and recovery. The use of the word partnership when describing the caregiver-patient relationship is a relative new trend. We now recognize that health restoration and recovery requires a collective, collaborative effort. Thus partnering is widely viewed as essential for clarity, trust, and cooperation–the heart of healing.

The provider patient relationship has evolved, with the caregiver taking on a more advisory role. Today's caregivers, in addition to being health experts, serve as coaches, navigators, and facilitators of decisions.

Although this book is for all healthcare professionals (i.e. doctors, advanced practice nurses, nurses, technologists, social workers, nutritionists and so on), a few comments about the doctor-patient relationship specifically are worth noting up front.

The doctor-patient relationship is a distinctive partnership with a common goal: make the patient better. The word *partnership* suggests that both parties exist on equal ground in formulating and executing a plan for the medical care of the patient. The doctor's role is to serve as an educator and adviser and to provide compassionate support. The patient's role is threefold: (1) to be honest and forthcoming in helping the doctor understand his or her symptoms, (2) to be involved in the discussion of various options, and (3) to let the doctor know his or her preferences after the pros and cons have been carefully explained. The patient and family, with guidance from the doctor, are engaged increasingly in decision-making and taking the reins in healthcare decisions.

Unfortunately many factors affect the caregiver-patient relationship, including time, continuity, personality, skills, environment, experience, circumstances, and beliefs. Because it is the physician who has the "prescriptive" power in this relationship, patients can be intimidated and, as a result, less than forthcoming. Some of the more common communications challenges that result from this dynamic are noted in Part I of this book.

With regard to caregivers who are not doctors, the same requirements for the relationship apply. Trust and full disclosure are essential. Interactions need to be laced with compassion and empathy to sustain personal respect and support healing–the common goal of all parties.

The caregiver-patient relationship works extremely well when both parties are willing to enter the relationship in good faith. It breaks down quickly when one or the other becomes authoritarian or manipulative. Friendship, concern, privacy, trust, empathy, and equality are all involved and should be carefully respected.

I wish I could say that all caregiver-patient relationships have these ideal characteristics. The good news is that with intention, skill development, and prompts, caregivers and patients alike can engage in communications that embrace these attributes and, in so doing, enhance healing.

The Role of Communications in Healing

Central to healing are the processes of gathering information, developing and maintaining a therapeutic partnership, and communicating information. These three functions inextricably interact. They form a critical teaching-learning process.

The essential processes of healing are (1) communication exchanges in which data are gathered, (2) diagnoses and treatment plans, (3) discussions and decisions, (4) adherence, (5) healing, patient activation, and support.

Caregivers tend to use a directive style of communications. They tell the patient what he or she needs to know. In turn patients (and their families) are more expressive. They need and ask for dialogue.

My doctor said –	The patient wants –
My nurse said –	The patient agreed to –
My therapist said –	The patient's family insists –
The social worker said –	The patient's wife asked –
The dietician said –	The family refuses –

Healing literally means "to make whole." It is the restoration of health to an unbalanced, diseased, or damaged organism. Healing may be physical or psychological. With respect to physical damage or disease, healing involves the repair of living tissue, organs and the biological system as a whole and resumption of normal functioning. Psychological healing enables a patient to resume a normal or fulfilling existence without being overwhelmed by psychopathological phenomena.

The quality of the relationship directly determines the completeness and quality of information elicited and understood. If the patient does not trust the doctor, he or she will not disclose complete information efficiently. Patients who are anxious will not comprehend information clearly, regardless of how often we go over the details with them. Thus the quality of the relationship also has a major influence on practitioner and patient satisfaction. In the long-term, high-quality relationships help prevent healthcare burnout and turnover for caregivers. For patients, effective communications is the major determinant of compliance.

> **Increasing data suggest that patients activated in the medical encounter to ask questions and to participate in their care do better biologically, enjoy a higher quality of life, and have higher satisfaction levels.**

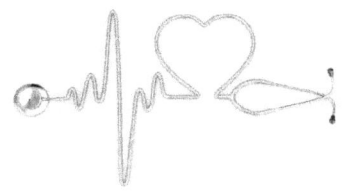

Part I
WHY HEALTHCARE COMMUNICATIONS BREAK DOWN

This book is all about healing conversations, and the argument for them is a strong one. Why, then, aren't we engaging patients in "healthy" dialogue on a regular basis? Several factors account for this: prevailing past practices, lack of skills from poor hiring and training practices, psychosocial dynamics, environmental factors, and relationship dynamics.

Part I presents six barriers to effective communications with patients and families. These are not given as excuses; rather, caregivers should become familiar with them, for failure to recognize and address these factors will hinder healing conversations.

Our challenge is to recognize what is happening in our relationship with the patient, and this includes realizing when communications break down.

Chapter 1
SO MANY PEOPLE!

Once when I was teaching a class on healthcare management, I had a wonderful aha moment.

Of the thirty graduate students in a healthcare management class I taught in 1990, only <u>three</u> had any experience even remotely related to health care. I wasn't sure how to make the material meaningful to them. I decided to create an example that would enable the class to appreciate the depth and scope of health care.

First I asked one of the students to feign illness, and then I asked him the first thing he might do upon becoming ill. His answer: "Go to the local pharmacy and get some drugs." I continued his story for him. Self-medication doesn't work, and so he makes an appointment with his family physician. The doctor orders blood work and X-rays and writes multiple prescriptions. Alas, the student patient is still not getting better—so his doctor admits him to the hospital. More specialists are called in. There are more tests, and numerous specialists are involved in interpreting the results.

I suggested that some problems were uncovered that required surgery to correct. Surgeons, anesthesiologists, respiratory therapists, specialty nurses, and physical therapists were now involved in his care and treatment. Social service had been consulted to identify any special needs or services important post discharge. Fortunately, the student patient did not require rehab, home care, or extensive follow-up outpatient treatment. He was discharged to home.

I used white-boards to map this healthcare journey—and noted on my timeline the various professionals engaged along the way and the occasions of billable transactions. I ended up filling four white-boards.

I then stood back and asked the class what they saw. From the back of the room, I heard someone exclaim: "A Lot of People!"

Health care is labor-intensive. Contrary to popular belief, advanced technology with high price tags is *not* the largest part of the budget in most healthcare organizations. Routinely, the cost of payroll is at least 60 percent of the operating budget.

Job directories cite close to fifty types of professionals/paraprofessionals engaged in healthcare delivery, not including professionals in finance, marketing, public relations, human resources, or spiritual care, or the tremendous support offered by housekeeping, maintenance, and dietary workers. Equipment vendors and drug representatives are also involved in treatment. In fact, as many as thirty different persons may administer services directly to a hospitalized patient in a single day. And this does not account for the countless others working behind the scenes before, during, and after the patient's stay. The sheer volume of contacts and handoffs is confusing for patients and families. It's also the source of major breakdowns in communications,—resulting in the diminished quality of care.

It is so critical for patients and their families to know who everyone is and what it is each person does. The arrival of white-boards in patients' rooms is a great start. But these only work if staff members use them regularly and expand on what is written on them. And some who have direct contact with patients are not routinely afforded space on the white-board (i.e., lab technicians, clergy, therapists, and social workers).

> **COMMUNICATIONS ESSENTIAL:**
>
> Healing conversations require clarity about who is doing what, and why.

With so many people engaged in the delivery of care, communications *among* caregivers is also critical. Vital Smarts, a well-known consulting group whose researchers wrote the bestselling book: *Crucial Conversations—Tools for Talking When Stakes Are High,* devoted a significant portion of its communications study to the healthcare industry. Some of their research was featured in a *Journal of Nursing* article called: "Silence Kills." In that work, the Vital Smarts authors note the devastation that can occur when caregivers lack the ability to communicate with one another. For instance, wrong site surgery happened when as many as seven different persons involved in preparing a patient for surgery—including the pharmacist, the sterile processing worker, the nurse, operating room technician, the transporter—sensed that something was amiss but failed to speak up. The patient ended up with a partial foot amputation when he was scheduled to have his tonsils removed!

In addition, opinions and priorities can vary tremendously among the various disciplines. Horizontal and vertical relationship abuse runs rampant among those engaged in healthcare services. Some of this conflict springs from the emotional overload and stress of having to be right and have all the answers. Robert Wicks, in his book *Riding the Dragon,* suggests that caregivers often fail to process or embrace their emotions.

Instead, many experience perpetual feelings of guilt, frustration, and futility.

The demand to be right consumes and overwhelms doctors, nurses,—and all caregivers. I often describe the role of the nurse using the following scenario: having three patients in respiratory distress at the same time, all requiring airway suctioning, and knowing which one to go to first. The oft quoted view that nurses "eat their young" is likely to be the result of their functioning in a high-risk work environment and also a by-product of feeling devalued. Due to these circumstances, nurses often do not tune in to the needs of inexperienced colleagues, which can lead to breakdowns in staff communications. All these factors ultimately affect the quality of patient care.

These esteem issues are attributed to the longstanding dominance of physicians. With their power to prescribe, physicians are in the driver's seat, and many are accustomed to having patients and staff defer to them—no matter what. All of this is in addition to the stress of the environment and the reality that seasoned professionals may withhold vital information.

The Blame Game

Caregivers of various disciplines have codes of practice that dictate professional limits and requirements. These codes create gaps in coverage and disputes over roles and responsibilities. When such disputes arise, workers may refuse to communicate or do so disrespectfully. Patients, family members, students, and co-workers may then experience the second-hand effects of these workplace conflicts. Blame eventually dominates conversations, which not only impedes effective communication but also frightens patients and their families.

Several years ago, my husband's chronic health issues led to prolonged bouts with sepsis. For the fourth time in less than three months, we were in the emergency room of a hospital where we had both received care in recent years. It was our preferred hospital simply because we'd many good experiences there.

This time Bruce's, blood pressure was very low, and he was in and out of consciousness. Lab tests would indicate the extent of the infection and determine whether or not he would be admitted.

I sat quietly in the corner while an emergency technician struggled to draw blood. I knew from personal experience that it can be a challenge, especially with shocky patients, to locate a vein large enough to draw the requisite amount of blood. I said nothing. About thirty minutes passed and I overheard the nurse tell the technician that the lab had called and needed another tube of blood.

As the technician proceeded to draw more blood, the nurse turned to me and, with strong eye contact, informed me, "We don't have a very good lab here."

Rather than offering a simple apology and letting me know of the need to draw more blood, this caregiver opted to blame others. She failed to appreciate that, in doing so, she added to my anxiety and frustration.

Discord and disharmony—especially deflecting blame—can destroy productive dialogue. As a result, discussions involving patients and family members simply don't happen as they should. Rather than focusing on what needs to be explained and what needs to be understood, caregivers become more concerned with who will have the final say. Few patients and families know their way around this highly charged environment.

The key then is to recognize when CLEAR communications is simply not happening and moving to ensure that we engage in the following:

- ◈ **C**onnect as people first.
- ◈ **L**isten to what's said and what's not said.
- ◈ **E**ngage in dialogue—a two-way exchange.
- ◈ **A**sk if you got things right.
- ◈ **R**espond rather than answer.

CHAPTER 2
THE "DECIDE, DETERMINE, AND DIRECT" MENTALITY

Establishing what's wrong, determining how best to treat abnormalities, and then ensuring that outcomes match the desired end—that's essentially what goes on in health care. The patient's help is needed to describe signs and symptoms, and the patient's cooperation is needed to take prescribed treatment or medicines. And now it is expected that an "empowered" patient will participate in decisions!

Health care partnering and accessible health information have shifted the role of the provider. No longer is he or she the sole expert. The final voice needs to be consensual. Thus discussions are important, and dialogue is critical. Needless to say, healing communication is essential.

Too often, conversations that allow patients to reveal private concerns, feelings, and long-term priorities are lacking. And that's unfortunate. A 2009 study of 2.4 million patients conducted by Press Ganey indicates that patients want their emotional needs addressed.

Physicians and other caregivers often view weighing the pros and cons of various treatment plans as their purview simply because they have scientific knowledge for assessing risk, and monitoring cause and effect.

True, informed consent before procedures and surgeries is designed to engage patients in decision making. The problem is that the "informed" part of the discussion, which the physician is obligated by policy to conduct, is often lacking. It is difficult for the patient to understand, let alone appreciate, options and risk. Timing is also an issue. Informed-consent discussions often occur just before a procedure, and by that time, the patient feels compelled to go along with the game plan.

Despite a national movement underway that advocates patients partnering with their physicians during the diagnosis and treatment phases, few of us—doctors, nurses and others— are comfortable with shared decision-making.

This lack of appreciation of the significant gap that exists between what is said and what is understood was evident in a hospital admission of my ninety-five-year-old stepfather two weeks prior to his death. He felt just awful: he couldn't eat and was extremely tired and out of sorts. He lived independently in an apartment within a large retirement complex. Since I lived out of state, I called the nurse in the retirement community's home care department to ask her to help. I reported that my stepfather seemed really out of sorts. She in turn arranged for him to be seen immediately by a family physician, who promptly admitted him to the hospital.

At the time, our family was small and scattered. My mother had been dead almost twenty years. I lived in a neighboring state with a handicapped spouse, and my brother lived states away with a very ill spouse. All the grandchildren lived in other states. None of us could get to our stepfather quickly. I spoke directly to a nurse at the hospital and explained our family situation and affirmed our interest in providing love and support and also our need for continual updating. I urged that I be notified of any change in condition or decisions made about his care. I heard nothing, and each time I talked with my stepfather, he said he didn't think they were doing anything for him. He still felt awful.

The "Decide, Determine, and Direct" Mentality

He had been in the hospital six days when the admission director of the retirement community's skilled rehab unit called the hospital to inquire about his discharge. It was at this time that we learned that the hospital had kept him as an outpatient. The case management department had determined that he didn't meet admission criteria and had arranged for my stepfather to be moved from admitted status to observation status. When I asked why he was kept so long if he did not qualify for admission, the answer was that the doctor felt he was too sick to leave. This situation was worsened by the fact that since my stepfather had not been officially admitted for an overnight stay of three days or more, he would not qualify for Medicare coverage for skilled rehab care. He would be subject to full private pay rates.

When I complained about not being notified so that I could explain to my father what was happening and discuss his options, the response was that the hospital had to deny admission status or risk allegations of Medicare fraud. And since my stepfather was oriented and agreed with (and signed) all necessary authorizations, they felt no obligation to speak to our family.

It broke my heart to know that my stepfather was left to wonder why his healthcare team at the hospital was not helping him. The following week, my stepfather's condition declined rapidly. He again needed a hospital. This time we chose a different one. He died four days later.

The saddest part for me was knowing that my stepfather felt helpless and uncared for in his final days. He also required pain medication and hydration for comfort which he did not receive. When I chatted with the skilled rehab staff, they informed me that the discharge note from the first hospital did not include any mention of my stepfather's diagnosis of bladder cancer, which had been made six months earlier. His death certificate stated that the cause of death was bladder cancer.

Despite the number of caregivers, not one held the conversation that organ failure was occurring. A physician at the second hospital finally opened a discussion that included the option of hospice care. My stepfather embraced this enthusiastically because his best friend had had a wonderful hospice experience for the six months leading up to his death.

My stepfather was shortchanged and denied the opportunity to live out his final weeks in a care environment better suited to his needs. He died peacefully in his sleep his first night in hospice.

So many conversations not held well and many not held at all! My stepfather relied on me to interpret what was happening. He did not know what questions to ask. *And I in turn was not given the opportunity to interpret for him.*

With a "trust me" attitude, and a sincere "I'll take good care of you" intention, health professionals often direct the course of treatment, seldom looking back to see if the patient is still on board. As such, the patient's reaction and responses are assessed through the lens of the caregiver. The patient's role is passive, and often his perceptions are discounted, his understanding unchecked.

Out of necessity there is a strong task orientation in health care. As result, we can easily lose sight of the fact that our routines are not necessarily known or understood by our patients. When we fail to explain even the simplest of activities, the uninformed patient assigns meaning to what is occurring and that meaning may be far from accurate.

Consider as an example the safety precaution of checking patients' name bands while asking them to state their birth date and name. This routine is a national patient safety goal to ensure the right treatment for the right patient at the right time.

The "Decide, Determine, and Direct" Mentality

My friend Mary Ann's elderly father was a patient for ten days in a large metropolitan hospital where she was human resources director. When she visited, she was very pleased with the care. Staff seemed attentive and to be doing everything according to policy. In fact, she was so impressed that she met with the nurse manager to express her appreciation and offered to come to his staff meeting to praise the staff.

As she was driving her father home after his stay, she talked to her father about the quality of his care. Her father said he was planning to give the hospital low ratings on the survey they always sent after a hospital stay.

Taken aback by his negative view of his care, Mary Ann asked her dad to explain. At this point in the story, it is helpful to note that Mary Ann's father was legally blind. He quickly filled in the blanks by explaining, "After all the time I was in that hospital—-what was it…ten days?—not one person bothered to learn my name. Whenever they did something for me, the nurses would ask me to tell them who I was."

The use of wristbands and other signs to signal safety concerns are common practice to staff. But we don't always explain the "why." It's no wonder patients don't realize the benefit to them of our safety precautions.

Here is one more example of inadequate communications. I asked another friend of mine after major heart surgery to talk about the quality of communication during his stay. He was quick to say that the staff were forthright and thorough. Then he paused and told this story.

After Les had had his heart surgery, the staff, without explanation, put an additional band on his wrist. He was up and about, ambulating as required, when he noticed this new wrist band and asked what it signified. He was told it alerted others that he was a "falls risk."

He was livid and tore off the wristband. He felt that being categorized as a falls risk meant he was feeble.

This brief episode may seem trivial. However, this patient was a highly educated engineer and would have readily understood the rationale behind the caregivers' actions. Had his caregivers simply held a healing conversation with Les, he would have never gotten so upset.

CHAPTER 3
UNCONSCIOUS INCOMPETENCE

A vast majority of healthcare personnel are superb clinicians with the best intentions. Our challenge is to recognize what is happening in our relationship with the patient and also realize when communications have broken down. Earlier I suggested that a strong task orientation can lead to caregivers' failure to notice the effect that their efforts are having on the patient. Two other factors can thwart the best of intentions: diversity and health literacy.

Diversity

When I use the term *diversity,* it is intended to encompass a range of factors: age, gender, lifestyle, race and ethnicity, culture, religion, socioeconomic class, and so on. And diverse preferences and behaviors apply to caregivers as well as patients. We all are socially conditioned over many years and by many experiences. This conditioning affects how we respond to life crises and other events that lead to suffering.

As healthcare relates to life and quality of living, spanning birth to death, diversity adds dimension and complexity to impressions, perspectives, preferences and communications. Wonderful examples of this can be drawn from stories compiled by Geri-Ann Galanti in *Caring for Patients from Different Cultures.* I highly recommend that readers add this book to their personal library. There are so many ways we misunderstand or fail to respond appropriately simply because we're of different mind-sets, cultures, beliefs, and the like.

During a seven-year stint when I was as an oncology nurse specialist, I had the opportunity to work with a highly skilled physician from India. He was an extremely caring individual. One afternoon he shared his shock and dismay upon learning that the husband of one of our patients, a woman whose breast cancer was rapidly advancing, was seeking a divorce. During illness, he insisted, people need to pull together. He said that in his culture the family—especially the spouse—takes on that responsibility.

I agreed that this was indeed a sad development but that we really didn't know the circumstances. I appreciated his perspective and suggested that his culture led him to a view of the union of marriage different from that of mainstream Americans. His marriage was arranged, whereas most American marriages are not. I really didn't have any data to support my assertion; nonetheless, I suggested that it might be easier for those responsible for choosing their mate to deselect their spouse. His response was that in his culture, love comes after marriage.

I tell this story simply because it suggests that our reactions to patients and families are influenced by our personal backgrounds, preferences, beliefs, and attitudes. Bias can get in the way of our serving the patient and family as they wish to be served.

Health Literacy

Health literacy—the ability to understand and appropriately use information about health—is another serious issue—one that represents a major barrier to communications. Patient Rights require caregivers to provide language interpretation and adequately inform their patients—about procedures, options, and services. The challenge is to provide explanations in ways that the patient understands.

The heart of the problem is often not the language spoken, but the words we use to describe or explain medical conditions. We can spend a lot of time talking to our patients without them understanding what is being said. It is estimated that 66 percent of people over sixty have a moderate to significant health literacy problem. The percentages for various minority populations are higher.

Consider the following list compiled by the American Medical Association Foundation and American Medical Association. These are medical terms that caregivers frequently use in their conversations with patients without further explanation or checking for understanding. Yet, they are often incomprehensible to patients and families.

analgesic	infertility
anti-Inflammatory	lateral
benign	lipids
carcinoma	menopause
cardiac problem	menses
cellulitis	oral
contraception	osteoporosis
enlarge	referral
heart failure	terminal
hypertension	toxic

COMMUNICATIONS ESSENTIAL:

To ensure healing, conversations must be meaningful– all parties must be heard and understood.

Chapter 4
THE "GOOD IS GOOD ENOUGH" MIND-SET

For too long, mediocrity in health care has been tolerated and sometimes defended. A refreshing departure from this passivity came about in 2004 when Donald Berwick, a doctor and the CEO of the Institute for Healthcare Improvement (IHI), had the courage to create the 100,000 Lives Campaign challenging hospitals across the United States to commit to proven practices that would save one hundred thousand or more lives.

IHI researchers, using the kinds of analytical tools used to assess the quality of cars coming off a production line, discovered that the defect rate in health care (percentage of things that go wrong or have less than ideal outcomes) was shocking—as high as 1 in 10. Many other industries managed to achieve performance at levels of one error in one thousand cases. Dr. Berwick knew that the high medical defect rate meant that tens of thousands of patients were dying every year unnecessarily.

Although he had no ability to force any changes on the industry, Dr. Berwick wasn't deterred. He knew that certain practices would save lives if they were followed without fail. On December 14, 2004, he gave a speech to a room full of hospital administrators at a large industry convention. He said, "Here is what I think we should do. I think we should save one hundred thousand lives. And I think we should do that by June fourteenth, two thousand six—nine a.m."

The crowd was astonished. The goal was daunting. But Berwick was determined and invited hospitals to sign on and pledge to adopt six very specific interventions to save lives. While hospital administrators agreed with the goal to save lives, they hesitated to admit a "defect rate."

Berwick knew he had to address the hospitals' squeamishness about admitting error. At his December 14 speech, he was joined by the mother of a girl who'd been killed by a medical error. She said, "I'm a little speechless, and I'm a little sad, because I know that if this campaign had been in place four or five years ago, that my Josie would be fine. But—I'm happy—I'm thrilled to be part of this because I know you can do it, because you *have* to do it."

How's that for a compelling call to action? There's more to this story.

IHI made a concerted effort to help healthcare teams across the nation embrace the new interventions. The friction in the system was substantial. Adopting the IHI interventions required hospitals to overcome decades of habits and routines. Many doctors were irritated by the new procedures, which they perceived as constricting. But the adopting hospitals achieved dramatic results, and their visible successes attracted more hospitals to join the campaign.

Eighteen months later, at the exact moment he'd promised to return—June 14, 2006, at nine a.m.--Berwick took the stage again to announce the results: hospitals that had enrolled in the 100,000 Lives campaign had collectively prevented an estimated 122,300 avoidable deaths, and as importantly, had begun to institutionalize new standards of care that would continue to save lives and improve health outcomes into the future.

The "Good is Good Enough" Mind-Set

Those of us engaged in healthcare intend to give patients the best of care. However, delivering on this commitment is complicated due to a long-standing tolerance of sub-par performance, the complexities associated with diagnosis and treatment, and the failure to hold folks accountable. For too long, merely good has been accepted as good enough.

The overwhelming responsibility to keep patients safe—to do no harm—can lead to compromise. If you look to the physician community, you'll find a long-standing practice of withholding criticism of colleagues. And among nurses and other caregivers, satisfaction with getting the job done— despite sometime horrendous work assignments, extreme time constraints, broken equipment, and staffing shortages— is rationalized as, "I did the best job I could."

A study of more than 6500 nurses and nurse managers conducted in 2010, again by the researchers of *Crucial Conversations*, builds on findings from the *Silence Kills* study. Safety tools and procedures fail due to "undiscuss-ables"—risks that are widely known, but not discussed.

This "silent treatment" refers to calculated decisions healthcare professionals make daily to *not* speak up when safety tools alert them to potential harm. People are concerned about dangerous shortcuts, incompetence, and disrespect—but they hold back.

Consider what would happen if 99 percent were good enough. According to the Institute for Healthcare Improvement:

- Twelve babies would be given to the wrong parents each day.
- Twenty-seven commercial planes would crash daily.
- Nearly 37,000 ATM errors would occur every hour.

Outcomes are markedly different when health care is delivered correctly 99.99966 percent of the time (which is performance reliability at the level of six sigma) versus 99 percent.

- Instead of 5000 incorrect surgical procedures per week, there would be only 1.7 per week.
- Instead of 200,000 wrong drug prescriptions per year, there would be only 68 per year.

Without a doubt, great performance leads to higher quality, improved safety, fewer complaints, loyal patients, more referrals, and a shining reputation. If what we do is exceptional, then we *earn* the trust and co-operation of the people we serve. We make a positive difference and feel pride in our contribution. We feel less stress and more job satisfaction as a result.

Getting to exceptional takes conscious planning and practice that is habit-building. It means no longer functioning on autopilot. It means refusing to do things the way we've always done them. At the core of exceptional communications is identifying the words and actions that make a *powerful and positive* difference.

> **COMMUNICATIONS ESSENTIAL:**
>
> Healing Communications place an emphasis on quality at all times.

Chapter 5
ANXIETY AT THE FOREFRONT

What is obvious is often overlooked. Getting ill, needing treatment, entering hospitals, going home, entering a long-term care facility—all are stressful and worrisome experiences. Even the excitement of having a baby causes anxiety for families. As caregivers, we have been conditioned to act calm, cool and collected, and in doing so we may fail to connect with patients—fail to let them know that anxiety is natural and that we will do everything possible to ensure comfort and safety.

When I was a staff nurse, I went to extremes so that my patients would never see me sweat. I thought it was my duty to be on top of my game at all times, weighing risk and firing away answers and responses—and never missing a beat. And to some degree, it is important that patients do not see their caregivers confused, or struggling with self-doubt. The problem is that if we stay rigidly on course, we do not convey *caring*. We are disengaged from our patients. And this failure to connect on a human level feeds patients' anxiety. It fractures effective communications. When we're task-oriented and to such extent that we ignore patient anxiety, we miss the boat.

One helpful technique, and one that I've taught as a coach with Language of Caring, is called anxiety mapping. In brief, it involves gathering information and insights from patients (and families) about their anxieties at each step of an encounter. Then caregivers create message points, or scripts, and specific processes that prevent or reduce anxiety at each identified stress point.

The classic example is an outpatient visit by a woman undergoing a routine mammogram. Most women have the same predictable thoughts, uncertainties, and underlying fears during their visit: How much clothing must I remove? Where can I keep my belongings? How long will it take? Will it hurt as much as last time? Will I get the results immediately and if not what does that mean? What does it mean when they ask me to wait until they process the films? *What if I have cancer?*

Studies have indicated that in patients getting a simple outpatient X-ray, at minimum, five significant stress points occur prior to the actual test. But caregivers along the way often consider this a routine and painless procedure. We fail to connect verbally with our patients in ways that might offer relief from their underlying anxiety. It must be our goal to reduce or prevent anxiety to the greatest extent possible.

> **COMMUNICATIONS ESSENTIAL:**
>
> **Healing happens when the patient's anxiety is prevented or reduced.**

CHAPTER 6
PATIENT BECOMES A DIAGNOSIS

The need to get things right in health care can impair the caregiver's vision of the patient and his or her experience. The rush for data—more test results—drives diagnoses and treatment decisions. Patients can lose their identity to a diagnosis or medical phenomenon.

For several years, I was an editor for a medical malpractice insurance company. We engaged in research to identify common themes in cases wherein patients sued their hospital and doctors. We found that mishaps and misdiagnoses seldom resulted from not ordering the appropriate test or procedure. Rather, these problems arose when caregivers failed to look at and listen to the patient.

Another common finding was sparring among caregivers. In their quest to pinpoint the medical condition, caregivers often made critical comments directed at other caregivers, and these comments were entered into the medical records of the patients who were challenging competence and seeking legal redress. These written entries indicated that staff members were at odds with one another when determining the full extent of the problem, not to mention the proper follow-up and treatment. The patient's voice was lost in a cacophony of caregivers clamoring to reach a diagnosis, make treatment decisions, and shift the blame away from themselves. *Seeing* the patient, and *hearing* the problem from the patient's perspective—these simple interactions were lost in the quest to "get it right."

Further, when petty disputes finally ended and the caregivers agreed on the proper diagnosis and magnitude of the problem, the patient's distinctive identity once again became secondary, this time to a label assigned to the disease or anomaly. Patients looking to lay blame if and when treatment failed, reported a lack of personal concern from the staff, that their identity was now lost to a diagnosis.

Caring communications is never simply about a diagnosis, or a disease. Once when my husband was critically ill and on a ventilator in an intensive care unit, I experienced the depersonalization that can occur.

My husband was unconscious and on a ventilator in a large academic medical center. A gaggle of physicians assigned to ICU cases gathered in the hall outside his room. As they conferred on Bruce's case, I watched their body language. All circled tightly. The physicians' heads were bowed, their backs facing my husband's room. Eventually they moved on as a group, with one apparently assigned to deal with me—the wife. The physician entered the room, but he never touched or even looked at Bruce. In a solemn tone, he announced, "Things are coming along. We'll know more in a few days." I realized that he was saying... "We'll know more, when we've had a chance to run more tests, and gather more data."

I wanted to scream, "Tell me about my husband after you have taken the time to look at him, or lay a hand on him! Ask me again about the nightmare we endured two days ago when he went into respiratory distress and had to be intubated and brought to the hospital in a helicopter! Ask me about what he was like before this incident. Inquire about our family, and what kind of support we're getting right now!"

Communications that heal are those that acknowledge that what is happening to a patient is most important, not the phenomenon of a disease process or medical syndrome. We need to keep it personal, and use words and actions that convey that we are intent, to the best of our abilities, to heal and restore Bruce, Mary, Jeff, Les, Barbara ... and all of their loved ones as well.

> **COMMUNICATIONS ESSENTIAL:**
>
> **Healing happens because the *patient* is the focus of all communications, and the state of his health is discussed in the context of the patient's own experience.**

Longstanding practices, complex decision-making, diversity, incompetence, a heavy reliance on interpreting data, not understanding people—many factors conspire to obliterate the best of intentions. Conversations become fragmented and depersonalized. Communications break down and healing is impaired. As caregivers, we must be aware of the challenges and take action.

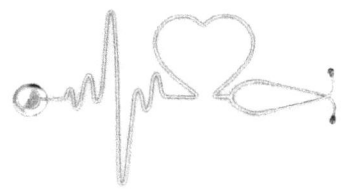

Part II
CAREGIVER-LED CONVERSATIONS: WHAT HELPS? WHAT HEALS?

What do patients want? Patients want us to address their needs and concerns. They want us to heal them.

Kenneth Haugk, PhD, of Stephen Ministries wrote a powerful book that I highly recommend: *Don't Sing Songs to a Heavy Heart*. He cites research conducted with over four thousand patients and caregivers, and lists major communications challenges in order of frequency.

1. knowing what to say to a hurting person
2. understanding, empathizing with, or validating someone's struggles
3. talking too much, listening too little
4. having a "fix-it" mentality
5. feeling discomfort in the face of someone's pain
6. focusing on self rather than the hurting person
7. wanting people to "get over it"
8. avoiding painful subjects
9. avoiding hurting persons
10. giving advice, being too directive
11. minimizing the significance of the pain or suffering
12. being judgmental

13. wanting to hear only the positive
14. responding with clichés, platitudes, or pat phrases
15. identifying too closely with the other's pain
16. feeling helpless
17. handling the anger of those who are suffering
18. knowing what would be intrusive or welcomed
19. getting people to open up.

After studying what works, and what doesn't, I've summarized the key principles for achieving healing conversations in a single figure:

CLEAR Communications

Essential Framework for Healing Conversations

◈ **Connect as people first**—Let others feel and experience your good intentions toward them.

◈ **Listen to what's said, and what's not said**—Understand that communications are complex and often veiled.

◈ **Engage in dialogue**—Allow an exchange of perspectives in an open, non-threatening environment.

◈ **Ask if you got things right**—Remain curious at all times, as to how well you've captured meanings and intent.

◈ **Respond, rather than answer**—Literal answers to questions are not as powerful as personalized responses to needs and concerns.

In the chapters that follow, these principles are featured in eight conversations, along with specific actions that help heal.

> Let Me Feel Your Caring
> Treat Me as I Want to be Treated
> Hear What I Don't Say
> Let Me Know What's What
> Help Me Feel Safe, Be Safe
> Let Me Know I'll Not Suffer
> Help Me Help My Family
> Tell Me What I Want to Know, When I'm Ready to Hear It

These topics, if addressed adequately, will enhance communications and improve healing. Caregivers need to first be prepared to have these conversations, and then make sure they happen.

Chapter 7
LET ME *FEEL* YOUR CARING

For the most part, those of us who work in health care do so because we want to help people. Those who stay in healthcare careers generally do so because of the satisfaction that comes from helping others.

Regardless of the circumstances, most caregivers work very hard to help their patients get well and stay in good health. The sad reality is that patients often do not "feel" our caring. Part of the problem is our intense task orientation and high risk work environment. Another problem is that we often do not have skills for communicating our caring.

Connecting with the Patient

So often the task orientation in healthcare leaves our patients feeling depersonalized. We're so busy ensuring that the right things are done at the right time that we fail to convey to patients and coworkers that their best interest is the intent of our actions. We fail to share the intent of our actions in a way that is understood and valued by others.

A critical communication skill is to verbally acknowledge or connect with the person at the beginning and the end of all conversations. This is much like beginning a sentence with a capital letter and ending with a period, but we are using words at both ends of the encounter to personalize the interaction. It is a simple but powerful technique. And these personalized communications need not be lengthy; they simply need to be sincere.

Connecting at the beginning of a conversation may be simply using the person's name or commenting on their appearance or behavior. Connecting at the end may be a sincere thank you for the opportunity to serve or it may be an invitation to ask for future help if needed. The critical factor is that it is personal.

Here are examples for use with patients or with co-workers:

> Connecting **at the beginning** of the conversation:
>
> *Hello, Mrs. Andrews. You look refreshed, like you had a good sleep.*
>
> *Mr. Miller, you are such a bright spot on my rounds.*
>
> *Sarah, I am so glad we're working together.*
>
> *Tom, you sound really frustrated.*
>
> *Samantha, welcome to our team. We're so glad you decided to accept a job with us.*
>
> Connecting **at the end** of the conversation:
>
> *I'm so glad you told me about your sleeping problems so we could do something to help you. I hope you will not hesitate to let me know if there is anything else troubling you.*

> *Please don't hesitate to let me know if you get behind and need my help.*
>
> *Tom, you're really an important member of our Team, and I certainly want to do what I can to brighten your day.*
>
> *Please let me know if you have questions. I want to help.*

Another technique that shows caring is to sit down when connecting with patients or their family members. Just the act of sitting shows that you have time to listen and hear what their needs are.

Our Nonverbal Communications Sometimes Speak Louder Than Words

Listening is another critical skill for caregivers. It, too, is a means of connecting with the patient and in a way that conveys empathy. As we listen we are also sending messages. This is why we often use the term *active listening*.

Studies indicate that the most impactful form of communications is visual—what people read based on our posture and facial expressions. This goes two ways. We need to tune in to what we're *seeing* as patients communicate, as well as realize that we are communicating our responses (stance, gesture, body language, verbal sounds, and so on). Patients and their families read caregivers all the time looking for answers. Often what they *see* shapes their interpretation of the caregiver's interest or caring.

Patients feel heard, understood, and respected when we *match* their emotional response. If moaning in pain, patients need to see us concerned, eager to offer pain relief. When worried, patients want some quiet time to frame their questions; they need to feel our quiet presence at the ready to help. A brisk, "Don't worry, everything will be alright" will simply escalate worries into annoyance and aggravation.

Demonstrating strong concern when one is overwrought is an effective gesture of empathy.

To understand how important the matching of energy levels is, think of a time when you were outraged at something, and the person next to you dispassionately asked, "What are you so upset about? This type of thing happens all the time." Your response was one of escalating anger, right?

Matching emotional responses is equally important in moments when one wishes to grieve or reflect. It is helpful if others don't push concerns aside with harsh directives that signal "Move on. Get over it." Kenneth Haugk, author of *Don't Sing Songs to a Heavy Heart,* warns against "pink thinking," which is trying to make things OK. Examples are:

- cheering people up.

- glossing over

- denial

- tough encouragement—buck up

- unbridled celebrating

I experienced the healing power of a healthcare worker who effectively matched my sense of urgency when my husband was suffering severe constipation.

My husband, Bruce, was a patient in an acute rehab unit. Having regular bowel movements had always been a problem for him, and during this hospital stay, the problem became worrisome. I mentioned to a nurse that it had been over three days since Bruce had had a bowel movement, and she responded, "Yes I know. It's noted in his chart." Two days later, I was again telling a nurse my concern, which by this time was escalating. Again, the response was matter of fact, "Yes it was mentioned in report." By day six, I was tense with worry.

A healthcare aide was chatting with my husband and me, and I mentioned to her my grave concerns about Bruce's going six days without a bowel movement. The aide stopped short, straightened her back, and responded with a resounding, "Well, that won't do! We'll just see about that." She marched out of the room, and returned shortly with two large glasses of prune juice from the microwave. She ordered Bruce to drink.

We had victory that very evening! Bruce had a bowel movement!

Our brains are wired to do a lightening analysis of faces from the time we are infants. We know that babies hone this innate skill by mimicking the facial expressions of their moms and dads and caretakers. Barbara Kerr, a friend and well-known expert on emotional intelligence, addressed the power of knowing and learning facial expressions in her blog post dated February 14, 2013. Kerr writes that our ability to accurately read faces as adults differs, but those of us who are more finely attuned to the meaning of subtle facial expressions are able to understand, empathize, and communicate better. She also points out that reading emotions in faces is a skill that can be learned.

Kerr also comments on the work of eminent psychologist, Dr. Paul Ekman, who has studied emotions for over forty years. Ekman developed a system, the Facial Action Coding System (FACS), through which people can learn to read the so-called micro expressions of some forty facial muscles. Ekman traveled into societies that had rarely, if ever, had communication with the outside world—to study facial expressions. His research led him to the conclusion that there are at least seven universal expressions. That is, if you go into any human society, anywhere on earth, people will recognize the emotion behind these seven universal expressions: joy, anger, sadness, surprise, fear, disgust, and contempt.

Ekman and his team teach doctors, lawyers, law enforcement personnel and performers to recognize these micro expressions, which can reveal "hidden" information about people, (whether they are being truthful, what they may be feeling, and so on). As we work with our patients it's important that we study their facial expressions for what is being communicated. In like manner, patients will observe us closely to get information about how things are progressing.

Acknowledging Feelings

An extension of nonverbal listening is the practice of acknowledging feelings. This requires us to verbalize what we are hearing, seeing, and sensing. Examples might be: "You look exhausted," "You seem down today," "You are especially quiet," "I hear a note of frustration in your voice."

Acknowledging feelings is an important way to demonstrate that we are really listening—tuning in—caring, and it often helps patients feel more comfortable disclosing what's on their minds.

A wonderful example of the power of acknowledging feelings occurred with Dorothy, one of my patients when I was a chemotherapy nurse. Dorothy was a quiet, refined single woman in her late fifties. She had been undergoing monthly chemotherapy for a lymphoma for six months.

On this particular day, I noticed that Dorothy was especially withdrawn. She appeared troubled. I commented, but Dorothy denied that anything was wrong. So I changed my approach: "What did the doctor say when he examined you?" I asked.

Dorothy replied, "He said I was doing well."

I then asked, "So why do you seem down today?"

Dorothy replied: "Last month the doctor said I was doing 'very' well!"

There it was—Dorothy's fear—her pit-in-the stomach worry. Had I not acknowledged her feeling, I wouldn't have been able to offer her reassurance, and she would have spent the next thirty days believing her cancer was back.

What if you're caring for someone who's lost significant weight or is suddenly bald as a result of his or her illness or treatment? What do you say that is supportive, and at the same time opens up the conversation for the patient to speak openly? Haugk, author of *Don't Sing Songs to a Heavy Heart*, offers three suggestions:

- *What is this like for you?*

- *I see that the condition has left some changes.*

- *I'm sorry you are facing this life change.*

We also need to allow our patients' humanity to surface. Each person has a distinctive take on life—we experience life through personal filters. The dynamics of family, personal belief systems, and past life experiences heavily influence a patient's personal response to illness and injury—they shape his or her healing potential.

As caregivers we need to gain insight and demonstrate respect for our patients' personal thinking, beliefs, and values. And we need to take it one step further. We need to convey our understanding and respect, and this is not always an easy thing to do. However, patients view caring people as those who make the effort to attend to their unspoken concerns in a way that says: *I understand that this matters to you.* This next story brings this home for me.

My mother's death was a sorrowful time. Since my father's death years before, my mother had been our sole parent. My brother, mother, and I had formed a tight bond, and this continued even after she remarried. My mother was especially close to my two daughters. Upon her death from breast cancer, I flew into "nurse, dutiful daughter" mode and began to take care of everyone. I helped my stepfather plan the funeral, gathered all family back to my mother's home, and delivered the eulogy. All the while, I never broke a sweat.

Years later, my elder daughter shared with me that it was important for her to see my grief when her grandmother died. I was so busy *taking care* of others that I failed to show how much the loss of my mother touched me personally. And my grieving daughter interpreted my behavior as coldness, a lack of caring for someone she loved dearly. I've not forgotten my daughter's sage advice. I now take time to share how much I care. I expose my vulnerability—I share my humanity.

It's really quite simple. Patients feel honored when you let them see a tear, when they feel your soft touch, when they witness you pausing to listen. This is the essence of making that human connection.

Saying "Sorry" Says You Care

Another powerful communications skill is a simple apology—one offered without making excuses or placing blame. An apology acknowledges that the other person experienced something that was less than ideal and conveys that you care about that person and what happened to him or her.

Examples of apologies include, *"I'm sorry that you had such a long wait," "I'm sorry that your news was disappointing," "I'm sorry you're having to go through all this,"* and *"I'm sorry that you didn't get the help you needed or expected."*

A blameless apology is one of the hardest things for many in health care to extend. Yet it is a very powerful way to connect with the patient.

When my ninety-five-year-old stepfather was held in a recovery room for five hours after a minor bladder procedure, he became **irate**. He later boasted that there were four hospital executives in that recovery room—due to the ruckus he created.

He said staff kept telling him they were waiting until a room was ready for him. They blamed the people on the inpatient unit. They also explained that they planned to open another floor to patients in several weeks, but at that time, they were pressed for rooms and staff. Staff gave me these same explanations when I later visited, even though I hadn't raised the subject. Though they were all quick to place blame and make excuses, my stepfather remarked that no one apologized for the situation.

Staff could have said: "I'm sorry about your long wait for a room. I know you want to settle in your room, and I want that for you. Right now we're waiting for the room to be cleaned and prepared." A simple, blameless apology would have made a world of difference. And my father would have *felt* caring from the staff.

There is power in the blameless apology. It lifts some of the weight and worry of a patient's (or a co-worker's) negative experience.

How Caregivers Can Take Action

- Connect with others by using personal words at the start and end of all conversations. Begin by using this practice in your e-mails. It will then become easier for you to apply this technique in your face-to-face interactions.

- Match your affect with that of your patients and coworkers. If something upsets them and they convey a sense of urgency, demonstrate your empathy by heightening the energy of your response to them.

- Acknowledge what you are observing, hearing, and intuiting. Check that you have the message right, and allow others to elaborate on what they are experiencing. This will open up lines of communication that you never realized needed to be opened.

- Recognize that a simple apology has amazing power. Make sure you are not making others scapegoats when things go wrong. Instead, simply apologize for any inconvenience, confusion, or delay, and take action to make things right.

> **Conversations that heal are ones in which the patient feels that you really care.**

Chapter 8
TREAT ME AS *I* WANT TO BE TREATED

Given our diverse world, the Golden Rule—Do unto others as you would want others to do unto you— has been replaced with the Platinum Rule: Do unto others as they would want you to do unto them.

How can you treat patients as they wish to be treated? Tune in to them. This skill is referred to as *presence* or the *practice of mindfulness*. Presence requires that we shift our bodies to a position of openness and readiness to listen. In this relaxed, open posture, the listener suspends all other thoughts and leans slightly toward the speaker—paying him or her full attention. While it is important to encourage the speaker with brief responses or slight gestures, we mainly demonstrate mindfulness by listening attentively to what the patient is saying. This includes noting the energy and emotions of the speaker. People who experience mindfulness report that they feel valued, that their opinions and feelings seem to matter to the other person.

While I was an oncology nurse specialist, there was a time when I struggled with remaining present with my patients. I had been in my job for close to seven years. My patients would report their reactions to the medicines, or comment about symptoms, and I found myself beginning to tune them out.

It was the winter of 1978. I was working in the oncology outpatient clinic of a large city hospital. My patients taught me a lot about life, the value we place on life, as well as the stigma and fear that living with cancer evokes. After seven years, I began to have trouble honoring my patients' experiences as they reported them to me. I found myself mentally disputing their personal stories. I had begun to stereotype my patients. I was not present with them, and I recognized this as a sign of burn-out. It was time for me to find other work.

When I coach oncology staff, I advise against directing patients' lives or prejudging what's important to a patient. Caregivers need to be present and allow the patient to live with their cancer as they see fit for achieving quality living. It is essential to get outside of oneself and one's own perceptions about how a suffering person should respond. Our focus needs to be on the patient rather than on what we believe he or she should think or feel.

Connecting with patients as distinct individuals requires a relationship of open disclosure. Patients will not disclose what matters most if they don't feel that their relationship with us is personal, respectful, and confidential. Patients need to feel that they can trust us to have their best interests at heart.

I'm convinced that most of us in health professions are kind, considerate individuals who have noble intentions. But sometimes these good intentions can damage a relationship. We make promises in haste to satisfy others. Keeping promises, even the simplest ones, is what establishes patient trust and thus encourages willingness on the part of our patients to tell us what they want, need, or desire.

My sister-in-law, Marie, underwent cardiac surgery in a large, reputable hospital in Atlanta. My brother, aware of my work with caregivers, paid close attention to their personal experience during Marie's stay. He cited example after example of the kindnesses of the staff, with one glaring exception: staff repeatedly made promises and then failed to deliver.

When the heart-shaped pillow that Marie used post-operatively to brace herself while coughing got ruined, the nurse said, "Don't worry. I'll get you another one." And she didn't.

When Marie's slipper socks got soaked and thrown in the trash, the caregiver remarked, "Don't worry. I'll bring you another pair." And she didn't.

When Marie's dentures were placed on the nightstand, staff assured my brother not to worry. They promised they would make sure she had her dentures when she woke up. My brother arrived and found Marie struggling to eat her lunch. Another promise not kept.

You may think these un-kept promises were little things but they added up, causing my brother and sister-in-law to feel disregarded.

Not keeping one's word erodes the relationship between caregiver and patient. It says, "I'll help you when and if I can remember to do so. Be content with what I offer to do whether or not I get around to doing it." A simple blameless apology is warranted when we fail to remember or follow through on a commitment. But a better solution is to follow through on your commitments to patients.

How Caregivers Can Take Action

- Ask patients and families what matters most to them.

- See what your powers of observation tell you as you look at the demeanor of your patient and his or her family.

- Inquire about customs and traditions.

- Know your personal biases, and make sure they don't adversely impact your interactions. Withhold judgment and seek understanding.

- Use terms that are universally understood. If you are unsure, check with your patients.

- Ask patients to tell you what was just explained and how it is important to them.

- Protect your credibility by keeping promises.

- Remember: if you have seen one patient, you have seen one patient.

> **The practice of mindfulness, or presence, enables patients to express what matters most; and the practice of keeping promises is essential to trust.**

CHAPTER 9
HEAR WHAT I DON'T SAY

A physician shared with me an important lesson he learned as an intern in emergency care. He said it was important to ask the patient, "How can I help you?" This question led to more candid responses than the traditional inquiry: "What's wrong?"

Often patients don't know how to express their concerns or what symptoms to share. They also may decide that the physician or nurse will give more weight to certain complaints, so they don't necessarily share what is of greatest concern. They might even share only those things they think will *impress* the caregiver. It can be hard to determine the real issues—symptoms and patient concerns.

To get to the core, it's helpful to use a simple question: "What is interfering with your quality of life?" Although this sounds vague, this simple inquiry often uncovers what is important to the patient. This approach opens the door for patients to disclose what's really worrying them.

To ensure that patients are heard, tune into them. Discovering the unique person within requires focused listening. Also it is helpful to use open-ended questions and "the five whys"—repeating "why" a minimum of five times. This technique helps you get to the heart of needs and concerns in conversations with patients and co-workers alike.

Here's what five-why open-ended questioning sounds like:

> Patient: *I really hate having to do all this therapy.*
> Caregiver: *Why do you hate the therapy?*
>
> Patient: *Oh, it's just so hard.*
> Caregiver: *Why is it hard?*
>
> Patient: *For one thing, I worry all the time about falling.*
> Caregiver: *Why do you think you'll fall?*
>
> Patient: *There's just no feeling in my left leg.*
> Caregiver: *Why else do you believe that you may fall?*
>
> Patient: *It's just that I don't think therapy is going to do any good.*
> Caregiver: *Why is it you think therapy is a waste of time and effort?*
>
> Patient: *My doctor told me there is a chance I'll never regain strength in my left leg—that I might not walk again.*

This is not the way this kind of conversation usually goes. Often we are quick to remind the patient that therapy is necessary to regain the ability to walk, that no matter how hard it is, therapy is essential to getting well. Thus we ignore—or never learn about—the patient's fear of falling and his fixation on a statement made by the physician early in his treatment. With careful probing, we can learn much more. We are then able to reframe our response in a more personal and helpful way. In the above example, the use of the five whys would enable the caregiver to explain the value of therapy in a context that has both purpose and meaning for the patient. The caregiver can also make a point of reassuring the patient that precautions are in place to eliminate the risk of falling.

How Caregivers Can Take Action

- As an experiment, apply five whys to a patient conversation, and see what you discover. Don't interrogate. Frame the why statement as a curiosity on your part.

- Share important discoveries about the patient's needs, desires and preferences with team members, either on the patient's profile, on the white-board, or in the written plan of care shared during reports.

- To discover your patient's top priorities, ask, "What is getting in the way of quality living for you?"

> **Open-ended questions enable the caregiver to help patients disclose their real concerns.**

CHAPTER 10
LET ME KNOW *WHAT'S* WHAT

While our routines as caregivers are familiar to us, they are not familiar to our patients. Patients need help to know what's going on and how it will benefit them. Often the purpose of even simple actions is not transparent to the patient.

Patients want to know who is who, and what is what. They also want to know what you want them to do. Families want to be briefed as well. Often we use brochures to explain things. And many nurses post signs to inform and forewarn patients and families. While these visual cues are helpful, they are not personal and can easily lead to confusion or misinterpretation. These approaches take for granted that patients and families can read and that they have their anxiety controlled well enough to absorb what they're reading. Engaging in face-to-face dialogue, asking encouraging questions, and checking for understanding—these are critical measures for ensuring that our patients and their families know what's what.

The caregiver relationship is greatly enhanced when the patient knows who is dealing with him, and why. When introducing yourself to patients (which is everyone's responsibility), offer your name, what it is you do, and, most importantly, how you intend to help them. Although color-coded uniforms and name badges help, patients want to know what you can and will do for them. Below are some examples:

Healing Conversations

Hello, Ms. Jones, I am Jane, your nurse for this evening. Your day nurse, Mary, did an excellent job of telling me all about your day. For the next twelve hours, I'll be the one bringing your medicines and checking on you regularly to see how you're doing. I'm here to answer any questions you may have about your care. I also will be checking on you to see if there is anything I can do to make you more comfortable. It is important that you help us help you. So please let me know if you need something for your pain or if you have questions about your care.

Good evening, Mrs. Winston. I'm John, your nurse. I just received a full report on you from Andrea. It's now my job for the next eight hours to make sure you know everything we are doing for you, and how these things will help speed your recovery. Part of that process is letting me know how you're feeling and what is helping. This is important information for me to share with your doctor. It helps us know if you're responding well to the treatment that's been prescribed for you. I also want to make sure your stay is a comfortable one, so please let me know if your pain returns.

Hi, Mrs. Williams. My name is Samantha. I am a healthcare associate. I work closely with your nurse, Andrew. I'm here to help you with all your personal needs. This includes such things as helping you with your meals and your bath, assisting you to the bathroom, and making your bed. I will be checking on you each hour, but you can reach me at any time by pushing this call light. I want you to let me know if and when you need help doing even the simplest of things.

Hello, Ms. Andrews. My name is Matt. I am the respiratory therapist, taking over for Lee, who worked with you closely through the night. I will be coming in to give you breathing treatments every three to four hours just like Lee did. I also will be suggesting some things you can do to improve your breathing both while you are in the hospital and when

> *you go home. Please feel free to share with me any problems you may be experiencing related to your breathing. Also, if there is something you've found that works better for you in terms of the timing of your treatments, be sure to let me know.*
>
> *Hello, Mr. Jackson. I am Dr. Davidson. I am a lung specialist. I, along with Dr. Franklin, who is the doctor in charge of your care, will be following you closely. I will be focused on the results of your chest X-rays, blood work, and breathing studies. I will monitor closely how well your lungs are working and suggest any additional treatment that you may need, from a breathing standpoint. You're in good hands with Dr. Franklin and I am happy to offer him support. I'll also be happy to go over the results of the lung studies we did this morning. I am particularly interested in any questions you may have about your breathing. I also want to describe what you can expect short and long term with regard to your lung capacity.*

A rich conversation is one in which the caregiver describes what is happening and why. You also want to engage the patient whenever possible, rather than just telling him or what you're doing and wanting him to do. Encourage patient input: ask the patient to help you help him or her. Of course you'll also want to begin and end all conversations by connecting with your patient on a personal level.

How Caregivers Can Take Action

- Make it a practice to hold important conversations that inform. Such conversations should include the following:

    - introductions that include your name and what you will be doing for and with the patient

- how to order food, when to expect it, and what to do if there is a problem

- the tests and treatments ordered for the day and how these will benefit the patient

- when to expect results, visits, discharge, procedures, and medications and who will provide these

- what to expect during a test or treatment, how much things will hurt (or not), and what will be done to make things as comfortable as possible

- when family members can visit and how they can obtain information

- any restrictions or suggestions about getting out of bed or going to the bathroom.

- how to operate the television, the phone, and the call light

- whom to talk to about any concern

> **Caregivers should not skimp on details about who's who, and what's what. Everything that's happening to, with, and in behalf of the patient is important to the patient.**

CHAPTER 11
HELP ME *FEEL* SAFE AND BE SAFE

Patients need to feel safe to express themselves and have their say. They also need to be free from worry about threats to their physical well-being and personal safety.

Regarding safety, first and foremost, the patients themselves need to have a voice and opportunities to contribute. Crucial Conversations training offered through Vitalsmarts is excellent for sharpening caregivers' communications skills in the art of dialogue. Dialogue is a requirement if we want patients to open up.

Several key areas emphasized in the training include:

1. Make it safe for people to contribute their ideas by noticing how people are acting. Are they being silent (avoiding or sugarcoating subjects), or violent (threatening, name calling, or using profanity)? If so, recognize this, and make every effort to restore safety. Two techniques recommended in the training are to offer an apology (e.g. "I'm sorry if I sounded ...") and use a contrasting statement (e.g. "I didn't mean to imply ..." "I simply wanted to ...").

2. Establish or restore the requirements for dialogue, which are mutual respect and mutual purpose. Mutual respect occurs when there is adult to adult communication (i.e., no talking down as a parent to child). Mutual purpose happens when the parties agree on what's important to everyone in the relationship and recognize

together that what each wants is not in conflict—that *everyone* is aiming for the same outcome.

Crucial Conversations training also includes ways to open and sustain dialogue:

- Use a "connect" statement to indicate a personal interest. (This can be as simple as using the person's name.)

- Note simply what you saw, heard, and observed. Stay factual.

- Offer what you believe you saw, heard or experienced. (This is your interpretation or the story that you told yourself as a result of what you heard, or observed.) And then ask if what you just offered is on track with how the patient sees things.

- Talk tentatively by remaining curious with your tone of voice.

- Allow and encourage ongoing dialogue by showing a willingness or eagerness to hear more.

- Close with a "connect" statement that reaffirms your personal interest.

Here's an example:

Mr. Miller, I noticed that you haven't been drinking your water. I am wondering if you're just forgetting to drink, if you're concerned with having to go to the bathroom so often, or if something else is keeping you from drinking the fluids we're bringing you. I'd really like to know what you think is happening here.

What do you think will help you drink more? This is important to your health, and I want to help you recover as quickly as possible. Getting you healthy is my primary concern, and I want to help you in a way that will make a difference for you.

Personal Safety

Personal safety is one of three things patients worry most about when hospitalized. They don't worry that caregivers are incompetent. They assume we know what we're doing and will act in their best interests. But patients worry a great deal about getting an infection.

Unfortunately, this fear is substantiated. Nosocomial or institutional-acquired infections occur at an alarming rate, and Medicare, and other insurers are now denying payment for care required to treat these types of infections.

Caregivers can greatly reduce patient anxiety by continually sharing with the patient what they are doing to ensure safety. For example, saying, "Let me first wash my hands, and then I'll be with you" and allowing the patients to see you dry your hands after washing them can be very reassuring.

Other explanations are similarly reassuring:
    "For your safety, we will ask you to repeat your name and birthday."
    "For your safety, I am putting up the side rails."
    "For your safety, I am asking that you ring the bell and allow us to help you to the bathroom."
    "For your safety, I want you to wear this special wristband. It reminds everyone that you are on medicines that could put you at risk for falling. It lets others know to offer you extra help getting in and out of bed."

How Caregivers Can Take Action

- Encourage your patients to ask questions, and seek clarification.

- Recognize when your patients are showing signs of discomfort about speaking up, and invite and encourage them to speak up.

- Advocate for your patients.

- Follow all safety rules consistently and inform your patients and their families when you are acting out of concern for their safety. Your words have power. Drawing attention to your actions allows patients and their family to see and understand that you are committed to keeping them safe.

- Wash your hands, and let patients see you do it. They certainly notice when you *don't* wash your hands!

- If the patient is undergoing a procedure for the first time, find ways to reassure him or her by sharing the strong credentials and experience of staff, the high volume of these procedures performed by the staff, and the expertise of his or her physician.

> **Patients need to see and hear that you are taking actions to ensure their safety. This will prevent or reduce their anxiety.**

CHAPTER 12
LET ME KNOW I'LL *NOT SUFFER*

It's no surprise that another top concern of patients in hospitals is ***pain.*** Patients worry that they will suffer. They also worry that we will not pay adequate attention to their suffering or that we will be slow in offering them medicine for relief. Waiting a long time for pain medicine is a reality that many patients recall vividly from previous hospitalizations.

Knowing that this is a common anxiety among patients, we need to go out of our way to let patients know of our positive intent to help them be as comfortable as possible. Then we must do all we can to prove reliable—to make sure they do receive pain medication in a timely manner.

Pain assessment is now part of everyone's patient-rounding script. Finding out how much pain the patient is having is simply an opening. The more important part of the communication is discussing what the caregiver intends to do and will do to manage discomfort at any level and early on. Most of us are familiar with the studies that indicate that pain is better managed if relieved near the onset of discomfort, and that if pain persists for a period of time, the memory is imprinted. This means that over time, patients will need more medication if they've had to wait out their discomfort, making prompt and adequate relief crucial.

In my discussions with caregivers, I've found some who fear that they may contribute to their patients becoming drug dependent. Another issue is that drug-dependent people do become patients, ones who require—and insist on—frequent medication. Regardless of a patient's history, if there is a disease, injury, or surgical procedure that normally triggers pain, we are obligated to offer as much relief as is safely possible.

Drugs are not the only comfort measures we can offer. Merely being there helping with a position change, or offering a cool cloth on the forehead, a soothing word, or a soft touch—are all actions we can take that communicate and deliver comfort.

Another comforting conversation is one that addresses emotional pain or distress by updating the patient on how things are progressing during a procedure or treatment. My dentist is great at this. As he works on my teeth, he continually mentions how well things are going. He expresses how pleased he is with the way things look, he reassures me that it won't be much longer, and he frequently checks if I am having pain. His check-ins and updates minimize my anxiety and ease my emotional discomfort.

How Caregivers Can Take Action

- Anticipate that a discussion of pain and discomfort is relevant for every patient.

- Check on the comfort level of your patients hourly at minimum.

- Withhold personal bias as you offer pain medication.

- Make the administration of pain meds a priority; ensure that your patients never wait for relief.

- Alleviate emotional pain, using skills that reduce anxiety and were covered earlier in this book.

- Reduce anxiety by offering reassurance and comfort continually to your patients as they undergo treatment.

> **In terms of conversations, caregivers need to reassure patients of their intentions and then act on their commitment to provide as much comfort as possible. Caregivers must be true to their word.**

CHAPTER 13
HELP *ME* *HELP* MY FAMILY

If you've seen one patient family, you've seen one patient family. It's important to figure out how best to help your patients *help* their families deal with the patient's health crisis. Generally we prefer having a family spokesperson, one who will spread the word to relatives. The patient should determine who will fill this role, and we should ask the patient how much information he or she wants us to share.

A colleague told this wonderful story about how to honor the needs of families:

Porfirio recalled the hospital admission when his father-in-law had open-heart surgery at a large academic medical center. As is custom in Puerto Rican culture, all his relatives appeared in the hospital lobby to pay their respect and support the patient's immediate family. Porfirio estimated that there were close to forty relatives present. The staff, recognizing how important family was to the healing process, arranged for space in a small auditorium, so that the surgeon could brief the entire family, following surgery.

It may seem apparent, but we need to ask our patients simple things such as, "Would you like me to tell your family about your treatment, your therapy, and your progress? How much would you like me to share?"

Sometimes patients want to spare their relatives. Other times, they want to include their relatives in all discussions. Some families insist that they bear all the news so as to spare the patient. This is tricky. The patient is the one who should determine what is acceptable. The point is to ask and to act accordingly. As the Patient Bill of Rights for Medicare Patients states, "Patients have the right to ask for the involvement and support of family." And in my view, they also have the right to deny family involvement.

Now to be honest, relationships can be complicated, and, at times, unhealthy. Some families are more difficult, especially when relatives are at odds with one another; some individuals may be at odds with the staff as well as they jockey for the position of spokesperson.

The bottom line is that we need to work directly with the patient to define how he or she would like to include the family and then support the patient throughout the experience. To ignore families is a disservice to the patients, and it complicates the healing process.

A word of caution: as caregivers, we might have biases that make it hard for us to tolerate, let alone accommodate, certain family dynamics. We may show this by going out of our way to limit our interactions with certain family members. Sometimes we also limit options and hide behind the argument that to accommodate one family member opens the door for chaos as other patients' family members will seek similar arrangements or accommodations. This occurred in a hospital where I served as chairperson of the diversity council.

I was talking with the nurse manager of a medical unit when a staff nurse approached. She asked if the adult son of a patient could stay overnight in the patient's room. I was shocked and dismayed to hear the manager's response: "We can't allow that. Everyone will want to do it." When I asked about the situation, the nurse manager told me that the patient was a ninety-year-old-blind man who was very ill. His only known relative was this son. I suggested that part of diversity calls for looking at this situation through the lens of the patient and family, and responding accordingly. I reminded the nurse manager that—one size doesn't always fit all.

How Caregivers Can Take Action

- See families as an important extension of the patient; withhold judgment of the dynamics you observe.

- Decide to engage families in the plan of care and then include them in discussions as the patient prefers.

- Listen closely to the family when they report that something is awry in the patient's behavior. Family members have important and helpful information.

- Continually inform the patient and family. Let them know what you're doing and why.

- Take the initiative to obtain copies of Geri-Ann Galanti's *Caring for Patients from Different Cultures*, and create discussion groups about the role of families in various cultures and how caregivers can best support them.

- Familiarize yourself with the cultural competency expectations of your organization and use these to guide how you help families heal collectively.

> **It is a great comfort to patients when they know that we're looking out for their families as well.**

CHAPTER 14
TELL ME WHAT I WANT TO KNOW, WHEN I'M READY TO HEAR IT.

The broad and varied menu of information now available to us on the Internet can be both a blessing and a curse. Even a cursory search turns up hundreds, if not thousands, of documents ranging from medical advice to personal stories and blogs about all types of diseases, treatment, and survival rates.

Patients often want to know what is happening inside their bodies. Reading or hearing about treatment options helps prepare patients for what they will go through. But reading or hearing about possible recurrence or survival rates can be too much.

Caregivers need to be careful to take cues from their patients regarding how much they want to know about a given subject. Not surprisingly, what patients want to know is often not what you expect. Nonetheless, they do want to know they have access to someone willing to hold conversations about how things are going and, if necessary.—about life and death.

Perhaps one of the trickiest aspects of our communications with patients involves discussions of prognosis. Many times full recovery is possible, and patients and their families want to and deserve to hear that optimistic prediction. Dealing with bad news is more difficult and the timing of such is critical. We need to deliver bad news according to the terms set forth by the patient or the patient's family.

What do I mean by this? Patients do want to know how things are progressing and expect caregivers to tell them. However I have found that patient's informational needs surface in spurts. That's why the oncologists I worked with were sensitive about pacing information. They insisted that all disclosures be honest, yet not brutal or fatalistic. They discussed prognoses in broad terms simply because we sometimes found patients who were told they had six months to live, lived well much longer. These Oncologists emphasized that no one is capable of determining time of death. They carefully dispensed information as the patient sought it out. They provided simple, honest updates, making sure to keep the door open to the possibility that things were not be as grim as they seemed at the moment. They allowed for hope.

Sometimes, we have to prompt the patient to shape the question that is on his or her mind. This may require several conversations over time. We need to listen closely and answer questions as the patient decides to pose them.

Twenty years ago, when my mother's health was failing, she asked my brother and me to come home for a visit. Her cancer was spreading and she wanted to make sure that we held the conversations we needed to have as a family. As we traveled after our visit, my brother and I compared experiences. My mother wanted to discuss her impending death with my brother. She pressed him to talk about his fears and concerns. With me, she never talked about her illness. She allowed me to help her with small things—to be her nurse. She chose not to speak to me about death or dying. I believe she thought that was an unnecessary conversation.

And often what the patient wants to talk about is not foremost in the caregiver's mind.

Tell Me What I Want to Know, When I'm Ready to Hear It.

My husband was diagnosed with multiple sclerosis (MS) during his late twenties. Twenty years into his illness, we attended a medical reception that featured information on the latest drugs and therapies for MS. At the time, my husband could still walk, but he needed a cane for support. The limitations of his illness were only starting to reveal themselves. The medical experts spent a lot of time poring over slides that showed neurological scarring common to MS, and they discussed how certain drugs attacked the disease. My husband said little, but I noticed that he wrote a question on an index card and did not pass it on to the doctors. On the way home, he shared his question with me: "What do I die from?"

This simple question often lingers in the back of the minds of patients and their families. Not only *when*, but *what* will cause my end, and what will it be like? Such questions present a wonderful opportunity to engage in a conversation that heals. The key is to listen and prepare for the questions, so that you can offer a genuine, empathetic response.

Another common question that often doesn't surface is: "What will I be able to do once I recover?" The key as a caregiver is to listen closely for the question and address the patient's need to know as it surfaces. Sometimes we need to clarify and prompt patients to make sure we heard precisely what they want to know, so that we don't tell them more than they want to know or what we think they ought to know.

How Caregivers Can Take Action

- Actively listen to what the patient wants to know.

- Prime the discussion by taking a guess at what might be the concern, and allow the patient to verify and expand.

- Ask the patient to tell you what's important and how you can help.

- If you are unsure or at odds with a colleague's perspective on the right thing to do in terms of disclosure, get a second—impartial—opinion.

> **The patient will lead you in discussions of life and death. Listen for the questions as they surface, and respond to those that are keeping the patient awake at night first, and then address whatever else is bothering him or her.**

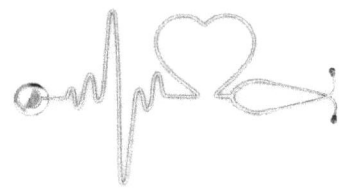

Part III
PRACTICES FOR CAREGIVERS AND PATIENTS THAT ENHANCE COMMUNICATION AND SPEED HEALING

This section reviews and spotlights behaviors that encourage healing conversations.

The appendix offers patient practices in a format that you can duplicate and hand directly to your patients. Some hospitals may decide to produce additional copies and make them available in waiting areas or the hospital's hospitality shop.

Chapter 15
CAREGIVER PRACTICES THAT SUPPORT HEALING CONVERSATIONS

I. Consider each patient and each illness—a unique opportunity.

Beware of this attitude: if you've seen one patient with gallbladder problems—you've seen all patients with gallbladder problems. This warning applies whether you're dealing with cancer, obesity, or any other condition.

I recall sitting in an emergency holding area of a large academic medical center and hearing staff ask, "Where's the PE?" I knew they were referring to me. I had multiple pulmonary emboli (PEs), and that's why I was being admitted. It really sounded cold to be referred to as a diagnosis.

During that same admission, I also heard staff talk about me in the corridor as "the patient with a history of obesity, peripheral vascular disease, and hypertension." Although all that was true, it was too clinical, almost hurtful, to be described this way. How about at least calling me by my name? It would've been heartening to be described as the mother of two adult children, a grandmother of four, a nurse with a doctorate in education, a former hospital executive, a woman who commuted over two hours to and from work each day for thirteen years, a woman with a keen sense of humor who was really caught off guard with this admission. It would have been heartening to hear some of these details about *me* in the information exchange between caregivers.

People can have identical (disease) states and yet their experiences and prognoses will not match. Many factors explain this. When I was an oncology nurse, I learned the value of not locking into a predictable pattern for patients with similar diagnoses. People simply sometimes live, when they should not. They persevere despite horrible odds. Others die when their death was not predicted as imminent.

My favorite bank teller, when she found out what I did in my consulting business, shared with me a book she found helpful while she was going through chemotherapy. Her husband bought her a copy of the *The End of Life Book Club*. (One of the book's recommendations: *The Etiquette of Illness* is also a good resource. I highly recommend both.) The point she wanted to make was this: "Sometimes while I was in treatment, I just wanted a day to pity myself, to be coddled. Other days, I was of a different mind-set and actively looking for ways to speed my recovery, overcome my health challenge."

It is important to know who the patient is in terms of values, fears, hopes, and expectations, and to know that this may vary from day to day, or even minute to minute. This means we must continually check in with our patients. Patients need to know they have an advocate and are not alone. They need a relationship with their caregivers that helps them write the best story of their experience that they possibly can.

There are two prompts that help us enter the patient's world:

- *Tell me what has happened to you as a result of the health problem you are experiencing?*

- *What would be helpful for us to know about you as we care for you?*

Responses to these questions need to be shared with others involved in the patient's care—not buried in the electronic medical record. Some folks use the white-board to capture some of these details. Others have notes that spark sharing during shift report.

How Caregivers Can Take Action:

- Listen to the conversations around you and personalize the discussion in terms of who the patient is and how this health crisis is affecting the patient.

- Refrain from categorizing people according to their disease.

- Communicate with each patient as though his or her story is the only one of significance to you.

II. Convey your caring attitude

One of the skills in Wendy Leebov's *Language of Caring* program is "explaining positive intent." This is simply telling the patient what you, the caregiver, want for the patient in the action that you are taking.

Caregivers who practice this skill are giving voice to their good intentions. One way to further strengthen this is to use the phrase "for you" whenever possible. When patients hear the caring intention, they don't have to just assume that you have their best interests at heart.

> The following are some examples of positive intent:
>
> - *I want to make sure that you are well prepared for your test.*
>
> - *I want you to be comfortable. Here's an extra pillow for you.*
>
> - *I don't want you to worry. Let me call the doctor for you.*
>
> - *I want you to be safe. Let me check this out for you with the physical therapist that set up your exercise plan.*
>
> - *I want to help you get a good night's rest.*

III. It's not about you.

A nurse once shared this story with me:

"My uncle had a health problem that required him to be hospitalized many times over many years. When he heard that I was going to be a nurse, he voiced strong disappointment. "Oh, don't become a nurse," he said. "All they do is complain to each other about their lives and tell you about all their problems!"

While this criticism may apply only to isolated experiences, it still raises an important point. As caregivers, we need to be present—and avoid self-indulgence. Our primary responsibility is to show empathy for the patient and his or her circumstance. Our communications should focus on the patient's interests, needs, and concerns.

And never—under any circumstances—should a caregiver lament to his or her patients about being short-staffed. This increases patients' anxiety and causes them to lose confidence in the entire team.

The only time it's appropriate to bring yourself into conversations with your patient is if you've had a similar procedure, diagnosis, or setback and can offer positive encouragement based on your experience. This needs to be done carefully, so as not to diminish the patient's unique circumstance. And it should be offered simply as comfort and encouragement (e.g. *"I know where you are, I've been there too."*).

> **A Rule of Thumb:**
>
> **Keep conversations positive, optimistic, and focused on the patient.**

IV. Families matter!

When I was teaching a session on conflict management to nursing students, I was disappointed to learn that their text cited the patient's family as a major source of conflict for nurses. Although families can sometimes complicate communications, more often, they simplify matters. Their involvement is critical, and families deserve our attention, compassion, and appreciation. We must see family members as our allies.

Why are family members sometimes upset or demanding? When people get sick or have a health concern, all those close to them are affected. Families are like mobiles. When an event touches one member, the other members are also set into motion. Parents of pediatric patients often feel guilty. They worry that they did something wrong or didn't do something they should have. And now their child is sick. Serving these family members can be a challenge; they might speak up in a way that strikes us as nitpicking or complaining.

The role of family member or partner can be unnerving and frustrating. Patients know when they are feeling better or worse, but family members must make guesses, and they often feel helpless. In order to ease their burden, we need to invite families into the healing process. Reframing our perspective might be necessary. We need to view family members as our allies in the healing process. Further the patient needs the support of family, and caregivers can and must help this happen.

> **An ideal conversation with family, updates and explains, and occurs in the presence of the patient. This enables everyone with a stake in the matter to ask for clarification.**

V. Play nice with others

Sadly, the blame game is alive and well in the healthcare arena. Conversations that include derogatory or faultfinding claims about others, especially among those engaged in the patient's care, can adversely affect the healing process. These hostile conversations increase the patient's anxieties and also threaten the patient's safety. Quality of care may also be compromised.

I once coached a patient care team that was struggling with negativity. Certain staff members continually (and loudly) complained about the organization, co-workers, working conditions, and more. This incessant negativity impeded teamwork. And further, patients were caught in the middle, overhearing these derogatory comments.

The team decided that certain team members needed to modify their behaviors and set down the expectation that no one would make derogatory comments in the presence of others. This was applied to each and every member of the team. If any team member slipped and began to make disparaging comments, the others would simply ask the offending coworker to "change the channel."

The team members also built in a reward system to celebrate when they had gone more than two days without anyone having to be reminded of the team's agreed upon behavior standard.

This approach worked for one work group, but every work group needs to explore behaviors and relationships that interfere with a healing environment and do something about it.

How Caregivers Can Take Action:

Here's how you can support the five practices highlighted above:

1. Rehearse the explanations of what you do and how you intend to help patients and co-workers. Practice this until it becomes a habit.

2. Bridge any gaps that may occur when others don't introduce themselves or clarify their roles and intentions.

3. Make it a practice not to complain, criticize, or condemn others at work. If you slip, find a way to change the subject. When you've eliminated this bad habit, reward yourself!

4. See the dignity and value of each person and enable all to be successful by appreciating what they add to the patient's experience. You can do this by giving simple feedback such as a comment on: what you heard them say (or saw them do), the positive effect their behavior had on the patient (or co-worker), followed by a personal word of thanks or appreciation.

Here's what that sounds like: "Mary, I heard you handle Mr. Augustine's demands in such a calm and caring way. He seemed to rest so much better after that. I know he is now much more cooperative with all of us. Thank you."

Reminder: Patients have enough to worry about. They should not have to worry about their caregivers' behaviors with one another.

CHAPTER 16
PATIENT PRACTICES THAT ENCOURAGE HEALING CONVERSATIONS

Even after years of working in the industry and being a caregiver (and later a caretaker of my sick husband)—I found my role as the patient or patient's family member daunting at times. Often I was intimidated and didn't say or do what I knew I should to get the best care possible. Nonetheless, over time, I became better at speaking up for myself and for family members.

Patients (and their families) are partners in the healthcare experience. Granted, patients are not wired to actively engage in the process. As caregivers, we must make an effort to identify and incorporate patient perceptions into the overall plan of care. We must also guide our patients to engage with us in healing conversations.

What follows are practices that you need to help your patients take on. Patients can act in their best interests, but we'll need to help them. Patients will require their caregivers support when asserting themselves into a healing conversation. The information guide that appears in the appendix is written for patients. It was developed expressly for caregivers to give to their patients.

I. Take Initiative. Speak up!

As caregivers, we are getting better at introducing ourselves and what it is we do—how and how much we are involved in the patient's care. However, sometimes we forget. And sometimes, our colleagues don't follow this practice. Patients may need to take the initiative to ensure this happens.

For example, if a physician walks into the patient's room, and states his name and the fact that he is a nephrologist asked by the patient's doctor to consult on the patient's condition, the patient (and, for that matter the family) deserves to know what nephrology means and why it's become necessary that the talk be focused on kidneys.

In like manner, if a respiratory therapist is visiting the patient for a treatment, it is important for the patient to know what helpful information to share with this caregiver. Namely, the therapist is not interested in the patient's bowel habits but would like to know that the patient has been experiencing shortness of breath with the slightest activity. How is a patient to know? The patient needs to ask! It is our responsibility as caregivers to encourage our patients to speak up—to take the initiative—to ask questions.

Here's what you might tell your patient to say:
Patient or Family Member: *What is it you need to know from me. How can I help you help me?*

If the patient is asked to agree to something or told something about his illness that he does not understand, caregivers need to encourage him or her to let them now. Also help your patient obtain a second opinion if he or she wants this to happen.

It is our responsibility to help the patient speak up. Patients need to feel comfortable asking for the space and time needed to digest what is happening to their health and to consider their options.

If the patient seems overwhelmed or uncertain, encourage him or her to let you know what would be helpful. Ask the patient if he or she would like your help in setting up another conversation.

II. Be Open. Communicate with candor

Whether adhering to an exercise, diet or drug plan, the patient plays a pivotal role in determining the outcome. Those with longstanding chronic health problems, experience little time spent under the direct supervision of healthcare providers. Patients may not know what's important to report, and yet it is critical that they are open—that they speak with candor.

Telling the doctor what's wrong is no simple task. Patients, especially those without medical knowledge, are often not sure what symptoms are relevant. They may dump a collection of problems or complaints, in no particular order. I was always surprised by what my husband decided to tell the doctor. Often it was not helpful; sometimes it was potentially misleading.

As caregivers, we need to help patients be clear, and it is especially important that they don't feel the need to hide things. Assure the patient that it is our job—to know what to eliminate first. Encourage them to report anything out of the ordinary—to be open about how they are feeling and what effects they have been experiencing from treatment.

> **Patient Reminder:** "If you have a hacking cough and have never had one before, let us know that. If there is a strange rash that appeared just prior to the cough, share that as well."

If a patient is uncomfortable with someone who has been called into the case, he or she needs to feel free to express this concern. The patient will need to know who on the caregiver team can and will help address the matter on his or her behalf.

Patients need to be able to rely on those caregivers with whom they are most comfortable—to help them communicate their concerns to everyone who needs to hear them, who needs to get the message.

III. Share What's Important to You

Sometimes when one is ill, priorities change. The circumstances can cloud what's possible, what's important. Knowing what one values most helps with decision making. I learned this when working with patients who had cancer diagnoses. Often, if I listened closely, I heard personal hopes and dreams that were realistic and achievable—despite advanced disease. I would hear of the desire to plant a spring garden, to attend a granddaughter's wedding, to visit with good friends, or to take a cruise. And in most instances, all these desires were within reason, they were possible.

Illness wins if the patient allows it to consume every moment, every thought. Concentrating on what one can do rather than what one can no longer do is really important.

A good place to start is to ask the patient what's most important to them right now. We can then work with the patient on what matters most to him or her.

Wendy Leebov offered up this story:

Here is a wonderful story of a woman who had degenerative bone disease and through the years had undergone numerous surgeries. She was at the point with her chronic orthopedic problems that one final surgery would determine whether she would become wheelchair bound. A close friend happened to be a patient advocate at the hospital where she was a patient. This friend came to visit the day before the scheduled operation. Realizing this was a significant milestone, the friend expressed her empathy and voiced her support.

The patient was quick to say: "I will live with whatever the outcome is. What will be is meant to be." She continued, "What I don't want to endure is the depersonalization that happens when you enter a hospital. I cannot stand being treated like a diagnosis….talked down to or worse, ignored by droves of physicians and nurses making their rounds."

The friend thought about what she heard and decided to act. She created a <u>six foot</u> high poster which she placed in the patient's room. The poster was filled with personal pictures and the following notations:

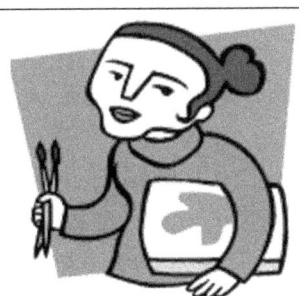

Dear Medical Staff and Employees
Re: Rebecca Roberts
- Intelligent creative artist
- Talented published writer
- Poet
- Magnificent human being
- X-rays show grossly positive sense of humor
- ALLERGY: Severe allergy to being treated as a child or a "hip"
- ANTIDOTE: Massive doses of sensitivity and care p.r.n.
- PROGNOSIS: *Strolling summer sunsets*

Caregivers need to encourage patients to talk about themselves. Helpful things for caregivers to know about their patients are details such as:

> » *I am a grandmother who watches my small grandchildren five days a week,*

- » I am an engineer who recently got back from an assignment in the middle east,
- » I am a widow who lives alone in a two story house where the bathroom is on the second floor and I am unable to manage stairs,
- » I am the primary caregiver for an ailing parent with dementia,
- » I am in the throes of a very messy divorce where the custody and care of children are at stake,
- » I am an avid sports enthusiast and miss playing golf every weekend,
- » I have lost a parent to suicide and another to alcoholism,
- » I am a devout Catholic or committed Atheist,
- » I am an art lover or the ultimate sports fan!!

> **Communication is enhanced when we know all parties in ways that help us discover what's relevant and what's not.**

IV. Speak from your heart

Honesty and forthrightness are ethical requirements of the patient and caregiver relationship. This means patients need to be sure to disclose what they are experiencing and what they want to hear in order for us to provide them the best care and experience. Earlier it was suggested that sometimes patients don't know what's important.

Speaking from the heart means sharing what is tugging on one's heart, adding to one's fears, keeping one awake at night. And this needs to be done using the words: *I am afraid that . . . I'm worried about . . .* or *I most fear that . . .*

During one of my husband's hospitalizations, I was so worried that no one would help him eat. He didn't look like he needed to be fed. But I knew that he often was too tired to put the spoon to his mouth, and so he would just pass on any food put before him. I also had been watching him waste away, and I had this horrible fear that he would starve to death. I knew without the proper nutrition, he would not have the strength to fight off infection.

I made an impassioned plea to his assigned nurse, and also the healthcare aid. But I took it one step further. I personally wrote on the whiteboard in his room: "Please feed patient!" Fortunately, Staff *heard* my fears, and Bruce received wonderful help and encouragement at every one of his mealtimes.

As caregivers we want to say or do the right thing. And that does include supporting our patients' emotional needs. The best approach is to encourage our patients to speak from their heart, to talk openly about their feelings:
Here's what I'm feeling. Here's what worries me most. This is what keeps me awake at night.
Without this key information, we can't know how to offer our patients the comfort they need.

V. Ask questions. Write things down.

Ask Me 3™ is a patient education program designed to promote communication between healthcare providers and their patients in order to improve health outcomes. The program encourages patients to understand the answers to three questions:

1. **What is my main problem?**

2. **What do I need to do?**

3. **Why is it important for me to do this?**

It is important that patients ask their physician these three simple but essential questions in every health care interaction. Nurses, doctors and therapists should encourage their patients to understand the answers to these questions. It is up to us to ensure that the patient is provided the opening and support necessary to have this conversation.

We also should encourage patients to keep a running list of their questions and to record the answers they receive. This way, they don't miss the opportunity to get the information they need, when they need it and as they want it.

CONCLUSION

Caregivers and patients need to hold conversations that heal. As caregivers, it is our responsibility to engage our patients in dialogue—in conversations that make a difference in their healing. Admittedly our role can be daunting, especially when dealing with people who are hurting. Kenneth Haugk in *"Don't Sing Songs to a Heavy Heart"* suggests four fall back practices for times we may have trouble finding words.

- The less said the better. Being present is what counts.

- Allow the person who's hurting to take the lead.

- It's OK to say, "I don't know what to say" or "I'm so sorry you're having this experience."

- It's OK to say, "I'm here with you—to support you all the way."

Everyone is capable of holding conversations that heal. It just takes simple know-how on the ways to bring comfort, convey caring, discover what's relevant and what's not, and engage our patients and their families in dialogue.

> **Caregivers, patients, and their families must be fully engaged for their conversations to be healing!**

REFERENCES

Galanti, Geri-Ann. *Caring for Patients from Different Cultures.* Philadelphia, PA: University of Pennsylvania Press, 2004.

Grenny, Joseph, Kerry Patterson, Ron McMillan, and Al Switzler. *Crucial Conversations: Tools for Talking When Stakes Are High.* Vital Smarts, LC, 2004.

Halpern, Susan P. *The Etiquette of Illness: What to Say When You Can't Find the Words.* New York: Bloomsbury, 2004.

Haugk, Kenneth C. *Don't Sing Songs to a Heavy Heart.* St. Louis: Stephen Ministries, 2004.

Schwalbe, Will. *The End of Your Life Book Club.* New York: Random House, 2012.

Wicks, Robert J. *Riding the Dragon.* Sorin Books, 2012.

A Patient's Guide to HEALING Conversations

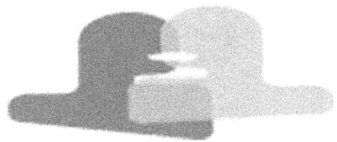

Dear Patient,

Those of us providing your care want to help you heal as quickly as possible. The quality of our conversations with you is important to your healing. Here are conversations you can introduce that will help us better help you!

Your Care Team

#1. *Speak up! Let us know if you are unclear on what's happening.*

If someone offers information or care and does not introduce himself or herself fully, feel free to speak up! If there is anything you don't understand or agree with, let us know. For example:

- ◈ If someone is in front of you and you have no idea who or why, simply say, **"What is it you do? Why were you asked to see**

me?" You may even ask for a card or for the person to write his or her name down for you.

◆ If you've been asked to agree to something you don't understand, simply say: **"I'm not sure what you're telling me. Please go over this again."**

◆ If you would like to check with your family before agreeing to treatment, simply say: **"I need some time to think about things."** or **"Would you please repeat what you just explained, when my family is here?"**

◆ If you want to ask for a second opinion, simply say: **"I am sure what you are telling me is correct. Still, it would be a comfort to me to have a second opinion. Can you or someone else help me with this?"**

> *#2 Be open. Tell your caregivers what life is like for you.*

Telling your doctor or nurse what's wrong is not always easy. You may not be sure which symptoms to mention. Don't worry about that. When talking to caregivers, just be clear and don't hide things. Your caregivers rely on you to be open about how things are for you. We can't do our job if we are missing pieces of the puzzle. Sometimes it helps to include a family member when telling your story. Family members can add important details.

Here are tips for these conversations:

- If you have a hacking cough and have never had one before, **say that.** If a strange rash appeared just before the cough, **share that as well.** Be as detailed as you can when talking with your doctors and nurses.

- If you're uncomfortable with someone who is assigned to you, share your concern with a nurse or doctor with whom you are comfortable. **Ask for help in finding a replacement, someone with whom you feel more at ease when talking about your health.**

The key is to communicate your health problems fully, so that everyone who needs to hear the information gets important details and you in turn get the best care possible.

> **#3 Know what matters most to you, and ask for what you need.**

Sometimes when we're ill, your priorities change. Sometimes it becomes unclear what's possible, and what's important. Illness wins if you allow it to consume your every moment and every thought.

Instead, concentrate on what you can do rather than what you can no longer do. Then communicate your hopes so that others can support you now and in the future.

- Knowing what's most important to you and then telling your caregivers helps with decision making. It might be as simple as needing help with your diet or bowel movements. Simply say,

"This is a quality of life issue for me. I would really appreciate help with this."

- ◈ Also let your caregivers know **who you are.** Here are the types of things nurses and doctors find helpful to know about their patients:

  - You are a grandmother who watches small grandchildren five days a week.

  - You are an engineer who recently returned from an assignment in Asia.

  - You are a widow who lives alone in a two-story house where the bathroom is on the second floor, and you can't manage stairs.

  - You are the full-time caretaker of an ailing parent who has dementia.

  - You are in the midst of a messy divorce in which the custody and care of children are at stake.

  - You have lost a parent to suicide and another to alcoholism.

You can improve communication between you and your caregivers by telling us about you and what's important to you. This information helps us decide together what's most important for your recovery.

> **#4. Speak from your heart.** *Let others know what worries you most.*

Your caregivers want to say and do the right thing. And they want to support your *emotional* needs.

Let us know what's tugging on your heart, generating your fears, and keeping you awake at night. Your caregivers want to understand, but they can't read your mind, so share your feelings:

- "I'm feeling . . ."
- "What worries me most is . . ."
- "What keeps me awake at night is . . ."

Without this key information, your caregivers can't know how to offer you the information, understanding, and comfort you need.

> **#5. Ask questions. Write things down.** *Take the lead in conversations.*

Ask Me 3™ is a national patient-education program designed to promote communication between healthcare professionals and their patients in order to improve health outcomes. The program encourages you as the patient to understand the answers to three questions:

- What is my main problem?
- What do I need to do?
- Why is it important for me to do this?

Ask your physician these three simple questions when he or she talks to you about your illness or treatment plan. Although your nurses, doctors, and therapists might think you understand, you may not be clear. Speak up. Also keep a running list of your questions. This way, you won't miss the chance to get the information you need, when you need and want it.

> *Your relationship with your caregiver is not one-sided. You have an important role in helping us provide you great care! We want you and your family to engage fully in conversations that help bring about healing!*

www.ingramcontent.com/pod-product-compliance
Lightning Source LLC
Chambersburg PA
CBHW051811170526
45167CB00005B/1968